Conquering Psoriasis
Your Comprehensive Guide to Natural and Medical Solutions

By

Denise D. Laird

Table of Contents

Conclusion

Chapter 1

Understanding Psoriasis

(What is psoriasis? Types of psoriasis, Risk Factors and Causes, and How Psoriasis Affects Your Body)

What is psoriasis?

An ongoing autoimmune skin disorder is psoriasis. Red, dry patches of thicker skin are the result of the rapid skin cell proliferation it induces. The rapid accumulation of skin cells is assumed to be the cause of dry flakes and skin scales.

This disorder develops when the immune system misinterprets a healthy skin cell for a pathogen and sends out erroneous signals that quicken the skin cells' development cycle.

Although there is no known cure for psoriasis, it can be controlled with several therapies. Although the precise etiology of psoriasis is unknown, it is thought to be connected to a problem with T cells and other white blood cells, known as neutrophils, in the body.

Plaque psoriasis, inverse psoriasis, guttate psoriasis, pustular psoriasis, and erythrodermic psoriasis are some of the several kinds of psoriasis. The severity of the symptoms and their variability from person to person.

<u>**Psoriasis types**</u>

Psoriasis comes in a variety of forms, each with its special symptoms and traits. Some of the most typical varieties are listed below:

1. About 80% to 90% of persons with psoriasis have the most prevalent kind, plaque psoriasis. Raised, red areas appear as a result, and they are coated in a scale-like accumulation that is silvery white. They can appear everywhere, but the scalp, knees, elbows, and lower back are where they most frequently do.

2. In children or young adults, guttate psoriasis frequently manifests as tiny,

dot-like lesions. It frequently starts pretty suddenly.

3. Inverse psoriasis: This type of psoriasis manifests as intensely red lesions in bodily crevasses, such as in the groin, armpit, or behind the knee. It might seem shiny and smooth.

4. Pustular Psoriasis: This uncommon type of disease is characterized by white pustules (blisters of noninfectious pus) encircled by red skin. On the hands, feet, or fingertips, it might appear in larger areas or more localized spots.

5. Erythrodermic psoriasis is a severe form of psoriasis that primarily affects the skin's surface. The skin could start to peel

off in sheets. It is extremely uncommon, appearing in only 3% of lifetime psoriasis sufferers. People who have unstable plaque psoriasis typically develop it.

Each of these categories has unique symptoms and can call for various therapies. Additionally, a person may develop more than one type of psoriasis or transition from one type to another.

Risk factors and the causes

While the precise etiology of psoriasis is unknown, it is believed to be connected to a problem with the immune system. What is known is as follows:

1. Immune system: Autoimmune diseases include psoriasis. This means that healthy

cells are wrongly attacked by the body's immune system. The fast overproduction of skin cells that results from this aberrant immune response in psoriasis results in recognizable plaques.

2. Genetics: The tendency of psoriasis to run in families points to a hereditary basis. Your risk of developing psoriasis increases if either of your parents has the condition, and it climbs yet further if both parents have it.

Regarding risk factors, several items can raise your likelihood of getting psoriasis or cause a flare-up if you already have it:

1. Family history: As previously noted, your risk is increased if one of your parents or siblings has psoriasis.

2. Viral and bacterial infections: Compared to those with robust immune systems, people with HIV are more prone to acquire psoriasis. Children and teenagers who frequently contract illnesses, particularly strep throat, may also be at higher risk.

3. High amounts of stress can affect the immune system and lead to an onset of psoriasis.

4. Obesity: Carrying around extra weight makes psoriasis more likely. Skin wrinkles and creases, which are more noticeable

in overweight people, are common sites for the development of plaques linked to all kinds of psoriasis.

5. Smoking: Smoking tobacco not only raises the risk of developing psoriasis, but it also might make the condition worse. Smoking might also contribute to the disease's early onset.

6. Heavy drinking: Heavy drinking can cause psoriasis flare-ups and hinder some therapies.

7. Some drugs, including some therapies for high blood pressure, heart disease, arthritis, mental health disorders, and malaria, have been linked to the development of psoriasis.

Though each of these is an established risk factor, having any combination of them does not ensure that you will acquire psoriasis. Many people who have many risk factors for the disease never get it, whereas others who have no known risk factors do. It is a complicated disorder with numerous underlying causes.

The Effects of Psoriasis on Your Body and Life

Although psoriasis is a skin ailment, it can have a profound impact on your whole quality of life and physical health. Psoriasis can have the following effects on your body and life:

<u>Physical Consequences</u>

1. Skin and Nails: The skin is where psoriasis most obviously manifests itself. It may result in thick, red patches of skin that are covered in silvery scales. The patches could itch or hurt. Psoriasis can occasionally also affect the nails, leading to discoloration, pitting, and irregular nail growth.

2. Joints: Psoriatic arthritis, which causes discomfort and swelling in the joints, can also occur in some psoriasis patients. Psoriatic arthritis may permanently harm joints if left untreated.

emotional and psychosocial effects

1. Stress and anxiety: Psoriasis's physical symptoms might cause these emotions. This may be brought on by the discomfort of the symptoms itself as well as a sense of insecurity regarding the way your skin looks.

2. Depression can result from the chronic nature of psoriasis, discomfort, and anxiety about one's appearance.

3. Social Isolation: Due to the obvious nature of the symptoms, some psoriasis sufferers may decide to withdraw from social situations to avoid awkward conversations or criticism.

Effects on lifestyle:

1. **Daily Routine**: Treating psoriasis can take a lot of time, including applying topical medications, going to phototherapy sessions, or scheduling doctor's appointments.

2. **Financial Burden**: For some people, the expense of therapies can be prohibitive. Additionally, if psoriasis symptoms are severe, they can make it difficult to work, which would increase financial stress.

3. **Lifestyle Changes**: Psoriasis sufferers frequently need to adjust their way of life to manage their symptoms. Changes in diet, a decrease in stress, abstaining from

certain triggers like alcohol and smoking, and increasing regular physical activity can all help.

The psoriasis experience varies from individual to person. While some people may only suffer minor symptoms that do not affect their day-to-day activities, others may struggle with severe symptoms that have a profound impact on their quality of life. If you have psoriasis, it's crucial to discuss any worries you may have with a healthcare professional.

Chapter 2

Psoriasis Diagnosis

(Psoriasis Symptoms, Medical Exams, and Diagnosis)

Psoriasis signs and symptoms

Although the signs and symptoms of psoriasis can differ greatly from person to person, skin changes are frequently one of them. Here are a few typical signs:

1. red Skin: These areas are frequently covered in thick, silvery scales. Although they can appear anywhere on the body, they are most frequently noticed on the scalp, lower back, elbows, and knees.

2. Small scaling lesions: Children are more likely to have these.

3. Cracked, dry skin: This can occasionally bleed.

4. Skin around the patches may experience itching, burning, or pain. In certain situations, the discomfort and itching might make it difficult to do simple tasks like walking or sleeping.

5. Nail alterations, such as thickened, pitted, or ridged nails, are frequent in psoriasis sufferers.

6. Joint swelling and stiffness: Psoriatic arthritis, which can lead to painful and

swollen joints, can also occur in some psoriasis sufferers.

The degree of psoriasis symptoms can range from minor to severe, and they might appear and disappear. They frequently go in cycles, with flare-ups (when symptoms worsen) alternating with clearing up or getting better periods for the skin. It's crucial to contact a doctor for a precise diagnosis and treatment plan if you have any psoriasis symptoms.

Tests and Diagnosis in Medicine

A doctor, frequently a dermatologist, will examine your skin, scalp, and nails physically to diagnose psoriasis. The typical steps are as follows:

1. **Physical examination**: The skin-affected regions will be examined by the doctor. The characteristic psoriasis symptoms, such as red, elevated patches of skin coated with silvery scales, will be looked for.

2. **Medical History**: Your symptoms, as well as any personal or family psoriasis history, will be discussed with the doctor. As these can occasionally precipitate psoriasis, they might also inquire about recent illnesses or new drugs.

3. **A biopsy** is when a doctor removes a small piece of skin to examine under a microscope. This can support the diagnosis and rule out any alternate conditions. Usually performed under local

anesthetic, this treatment produces little discomfort.

Psoriasis cannot be diagnosed with a blood test, and without a biopsy, it can occasionally be challenging to distinguish it from other skin conditions like eczema. Remember, it's crucial to see a healthcare professional for an appropriate diagnosis and treatment plan if you feel you have psoriasis.

Chapter 3

Psoriasis Medical Treatments

(Topical Medicine, Medications for the Whole Body, Biologics, and Light Therapy)

Topical Medicine

The initial line of psoriasis treatment is frequently topical medications. For situations of more severe psoriasis, they can be used with other treatments or used alone in mild to moderate symptoms. Here are some popular topical psoriasis treatments:

1. **Topical corticosteroids**: These are the most popular psoriasis treatments.

Both inflammation and irritation are reduced by them. The kind that is given will depend on the plaques' location and thickness because they come in different strengths.

2. **Vitamin D analogs**: These artificial forms of vitamin D inhibit the proliferation of skin cells. Calcipotriene (Dovonex) and calcitriol (Vectical) are two examples.

3. **Tazarotene** (Tazorac, Avage), a topical retinoid, can help reduce the rate of skin cell development. It could irritate the skin and make people more sensitive to the sun.

4. **Anthralin**: This drug aids in smoothing the skin by removing scales and slowing

the formation of new skin cells. Although it might irritate the skin, it is frequently used with other therapies.

5. **Tacrolimus (Protopic) and pimecrolimus (Elidel)**: Two topical calcineurin inhibitors, lessen inflammation and plaque development. They are typically applied to thin-skinned areas, such as the area around the eyes, where steroid creams would put the skin in too great a danger of weakening.

6. **Salicylic acid**: Encourages the shedding of psoriatic scales and is available over-the-counter (OTC) and by prescription.

7. **Coal tar**, a byproduct of the processing of coal, can lessen symptoms and decrease the rapid proliferation of skin cells. It is sold over the counter in a variety of goods, including shampoos, lotions, and oils.

It's crucial to keep in mind that every person's skin responds to these treatments differently. Finding the most efficient course of treatment frequently requires trial and error because what works for one person may not work for another. Before beginning a new treatment regimen, always check with a healthcare professional.

<u>Systems-wide Medications</u>

Drugs that operate systemically are those that affect the entire body. They are typically prescribed for those with mild to moderate psoriasis, or psoriatic arthritis, or for people who don't respond to topical medications or UV light therapy. Here are some examples of frequently used systemic drugs:

1. **Methotrexate**: This medication can aid in reducing the generation of new skin cells and reducing inflammation. Psoriatic arthritis can also be effectively treated with it.

2. **Cyclosporine**: This immunosuppressive drug works similarly to methotrexate in suppressing the

immune system. Because of possible negative side effects including renal damage and high blood pressure, it is often only taken for brief periods.

3. **Retinoids**: These are substances that resemble vitamin A in their characteristics. When other treatments are ineffective for severe cases, acitretin (Soriatane) can be extremely beneficial.

4. **Biologics**: These medications target particular immune system organs. They include drugs like etanercept (Enbrel), infliximab (Remicade), adalimumab (Humira), ustekinumab (Stelara), secukinumab (Cosentyx), and ixekizumab (Taltz), and are typically administered via injection.

5. **PDE4 inhibitors**: A relatively new family of medications, apremilast (Otezla), works by decreasing inflammation.

6. **JAK inhibitors** are a relatively recent class of medications that work by inhibiting the activity of one or more members of the Janus kinase family of enzymes to stop the inflammatory immune response. Xeljanz's tofacitinib is one illustration.

Systemic drugs are frequently used for brief periods and may be alternated with other forms of treatment because they can be extremely effective but also have possible negative effects. When utilizing these medicines, it's important to follow up frequently with your doctor to check for any negative side effects.

Luminous therapy

Psoriasis patients may benefit from light therapy, sometimes referred to as phototherapy, which includes exposing the skin to ultraviolet (UV) light while under a doctor's care. Several types of light treatment for psoriasis include the following:

1. **UVB Phototherapy**: One popular type of phototherapy for the treatment of psoriasis uses UVB light. It can be administered topically alone or in conjunction with other drugs. Using a

UVB lamp, UVB phototherapy can be carried out in a doctor's office or at home.

2. Using a **narrower band** of the UVB spectrum, narrow-band UVB therapy is a more recent type of phototherapy. It works just as well as broadband UVB and frequently more swiftly. But it can also result in burns that are more severe and stay longer.

3. The **psoralen plus ultraviolet** A (PUVA) therapy involves taking a light-sensitizing drug (psoralen) before being exposed to UVA light. Psoralen increases the skin's receptivity to UVA exposure, which penetrates the skin more deeply than UVB rays. For more severe cases of psoriasis, this more rigorous

treatment is frequently utilized and consistently improves skin.

4. **Excimer laser**: This type of light therapy targets only the affected skin and is used to treat mild to moderate psoriasis. To help with the reduction of inflammation and excessive skin cell formation, a controlled beam of UVB radiation at a certain wavelength is focused on the area affected by psoriasis.

5. **Pulsed dye laser**: This kind of light therapy destroys the minute blood vessels that cause psoriatic plaques by using a different kind of light.

Some of the dangers associated with sun exposure, such as skin aging and an increased risk of skin cancer, are also present in light treatment. It necessitates time commitment and could not be insured. To determine whether light therapy is an appropriate option for you depending on your unique illness, lifestyle, and general health, it is always advisable to speak with a healthcare professional.

Chapter 4

Psoriasis Natural Treatments

(Dietary adjustments, dietary supplements, mind-body treatments, herbal remedies)

There is no known cure for psoriasis, however, certain natural therapies may help you manage your symptoms or support your doctor's recommended treatment strategy. Always remember that before attempting things, you should talk about them with your doctor. Here are a few possibilities:

1. **Aloe Vera**: When used topically, aloe vera may lessen the psoriasis-related redness and scaling.

2. **Fish oil**: Though research is conflicting, taking fish oil supplements that are high in omega-3 fatty acids may help reduce inflammation.

3. **Turmeric**: According to some research, applying or ingesting turmeric topically or internally may help to lessen psoriasis flare-ups.

4. **Dead Sea Salts**: Soaking in a warm bath (not hot) with Dead Sea salts or Epsom salts added can help remove scales and reduce irritation.

5. According to certain research, **topical creams** containing 10% Oregon grape (Mahonia Aquifolium) may aid in the treatment of mild to moderate psoriasis.

6. **Tea tree oil**: Tea tree oil can be calming to the skin and is known to have antiseptic properties. Some people discover that using shampoos containing tea tree oil relieves the psoriasis on their scalp.

7. **Meditation and Stress Reduction Methods**: Because stress can cause psoriasis flare-ups, methods like breathing exercises, yoga, and meditation can help you control your stress levels.

8. No specific diet is known to help with psoriasis, although eating well can still be helpful. When they cut down on dairy and gluten, some people find that their symptoms become better. Keeping a meal journal can be useful for identifying any potential triggers.

Keep in mind that what functions for one individual may not function for another. To ascertain the success of several of these treatments, more research is required. Before beginning any natural cure, it's important to speak with a healthcare professional because some of them may conflict with your existing treatment or produce negative effects.

Chapter 5

Living with Psoriasis

(Dealing with Flare-Ups, Emotional and Stress Management, and Skin Care Advice)

Managing Flare-Ups

Flare-ups of psoriasis can be difficult to treat, however, some methods work:

1. Even if you are not currently suffering a flare-up, it is important to follow the treatment plan recommended by your healthcare physician. Future flare-ups may become less frequent and less severe as a result of this.

2. Determine Triggers: Many psoriasis sufferers have triggers that might cause an outbreak. Stress, specific drugs, skin traumas, and certain illnesses are typical triggers. To keep note of your flare-ups and potential triggers, keep a journal.

I'm make to lessen flare-ups and enhance your general health:

1. Maintain a Healthy Weight: Psoriasis sufferers are more likely to be obese, and obesity itself is a risk factor for the condition. If you are overweight, losing weight could ease your psoriasis symptoms.

2. Eating a balanced diet high in fruits, vegetables, whole grains, and lean

proteins helps boost general health and may help control psoriasis, even though there is no specific diet for the condition. Eliminating dairy, gluten, and several other foods seems to help some people.

3. Regular physical exercise helps you manage your weight, lower inflammation, and improve your mood, all of which are advantageous for persons with psoriasis.

4. Limit Alcohol Consumption: Alcohol may reduce the efficacy of some psoriasis therapies and cause psoriasis flare-ups.

5. Quit Smoking: Psoriasis is more likely if you smoke. Additionally, it can exacerbate your symptoms if you already have psoriasis.

6. Stress reduction: Stress can cause flare-ups of psoriasis. Deep breathing, yoga, meditation, and other stress-reduction methods can be helpful.

7. Regular Sleep: Good sleep is essential for maintaining overall health and helps reduce stress. Create a relaxing setting for sleeping and attempt to establish a regular sleep pattern.

8. Drink enough water to keep your skin hydrated and perhaps lessen the symptoms of psoriasis.

Always remember to speak with your doctor before making any major lifestyle adjustments, especially if you have other medical issues. Your healthcare practitioner can offer advice based on your unique circumstances and need.

Environmental Elements

Psoriasis can be greatly impacted by environmental conditions, which can lead to flare-ups or exacerbate symptoms. Here are a few to think about:

1. Weather: Dry, chilly conditions can dry up your skin and aggravate psoriasis. On the other hand, warm, bright weather can help alleviate the symptoms of psoriasis since sunlight helps lessen swelling and delay the overproduction of skin cells which is typical of psoriasis.

2. Stress: A psoriasis flare can be brought on by stressful situations or by extended periods of stress. For this reason, stress reduction tactics can be helpful for psoriasis sufferers.

3. Skin Trauma: The Koebner phenomenon describes how physical harm to the skin, such as a cut, scrape, bug bite, or sunburn, can cause psoriasis to flare up.

4. Diseases: Particularly in children and young people, some diseases, such as strep throat or skin infections, can cause flares of psoriasis.

5. Medication: Some medicines, such as those for high blood pressure, heart

disease, and depression, can either cause a flare-up of psoriasis or exacerbate it.

6. Substance Abuse: Smoking and binge drinking can both cause psoriasis flare-ups and reduce the effectiveness of therapies.

You can control your psoriasis more effectively if you are aware of these environmental influences. To find probable triggers, it may be helpful to keep a log of your psoriasis symptoms and any associated environmental circumstances. Always collaborate with your healthcare professional to create the best management strategy for your case.

Conclusion

A long-term, inflammatory skin disorder called psoriasis is marked by red, flaky skin patches. There are numerous therapeutic options available to manage symptoms and enhance the quality of life, even though it can be difficult to live with. Topical creams, ingested pharmaceuticals, light therapy, as well as herbal cures, and dietary modifications, can all be used as treatments.

Nevertheless, psoriasis affects people differently. Working closely with a healthcare professional is vital to create a unique treatment plan because what works for one person might not work for another. Understanding the causes and making lifestyle changes can help manage this illness to a great extent.

Given that psoriasis can have serious psychological effects, it's also crucial to manage stress and preserve emotional stability. You are not alone if you have psoriasis, so keep that in mind. You can find tools and support groups to guide you through your journey with this ailment.

More than just a physical ailment, psoriasis has a profound effect on many facets of life. However, it may be properly treated, enabling those who have psoriasis to lead a healthy and fulfilling life with the right care, information, and support.